Pelvic Floor Yoga for Women

Simple Step-by-Step Exercises to Address Incontinence, Prolapse, and Vaginal Health

Mandy Norris

Table of Contents

Chapter 1: Introduction

My mom, like many women, overcame the trials of childbirth and the subtle transitions of aging with grace and fortitude. Yet, behind the surface, she bore the silent weight of pelvic floor dysfunction. Occasional leaks amid laughing or activity, a persistent sensation of heaviness, and a calm acceptance of these changes had become her usual.

Then, she found pelvic floor yoga.

At first, the idea seemed daunting. Yoga? At her age? But with gentle encouragement, she went onto the mat, going on a journey that would alter not just her physical health but also her soul.

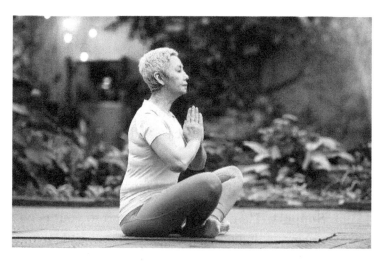

Practicing yoga

Through conscious movement and breath, she started to reconnect with her body, uncovering muscles she hadn't felt in years. The moderate flows and focused postures brought strength and flexibility back to her pelvic floor, eventually regaining control and confidence.

But the benefits extended far beyond the physical.

As she trained, a sensation of serenity and empowerment flowed over her. The peaceful periods of meditation on the mat encouraged her to release tension and embrace self-acceptance. Her laughing grew unfettered, her movements more fluid, and her spirit soared.

Understanding the Pelvic Floor: Anatomy, Function, and Common Issues

The pelvic floor, sometimes referred to as the "unsung hero" of the body, is a complex network of muscles, ligaments, and connective tissues that creates a supporting hammock at the base of your pelvis. Imagine it as a dynamic trampoline, reaching from your pubic bone at the front to your tailbone at the rear, and spanning the area between your sitting bones.

These muscles have several critical functions:

1) **Support:** They give crucial support to your pelvic organs, including your bladder, uterus, and rectum, maintaining them in their right places.

2) **Control:** They assist you maintain continence by regulating the opening and closure of your urethra, anus, and vagina.

3) **Sexual Function:** They contribute to sexual pleasure and feeling.

4) **Stability:** They support your pelvis and spine by working in tandem with your core muscles.

When Things Go Wrong: Common Pelvic Floor Issues

Unfortunately, the pelvic floor is vulnerable to failure owing to different circumstances such as childbirth, age, hormonal changes, surgery, persistent constipation, and even stress. When these muscles become weak, tight, or uncoordinated, a variety of disorders may arise:

+ **Urinary Incontinence:** Leaking pee when you cough, sneeze, laugh, or exercise.

+ **Fecal Incontinence:** Difficulty regulating bowel motions.

+ **Pelvic Organ Prolapse:** A condition when one or more pelvic organs slip down into the vagina.

+ **Sexual Dysfunction:** Pain during intercourse, diminished feeling, or trouble obtaining orgasm.

+ **Pelvic discomfort:** Chronic discomfort in the lower abdomen, back, or pelvic area.

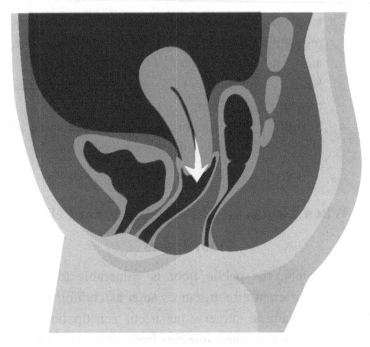

Uterine Prolapse

The Mind-Body Connection: Yoga's Role in Pelvic Health

While traditional therapies like physical therapy and medication may be successful, yoga provides a comprehensive approach to pelvic health that treats both the physical and emotional components of pelvic floor dysfunction.

Awareness and Connection: Yoga helps you become more aware of your body and establish a connection with your pelvic floor muscles. Many women are unaware of these muscles or fail to activate them effectively. Yoga positions and breathing methods may educate you to separate and regulate these muscles, boosting their strength and coordination.

Strength and Flexibility: Yoga provides a broad variety of positions that strengthen and extend the pelvic floor muscles, encouraging optimum function. By strengthening muscular tone and flexibility, you may increase support for your pelvic organs and lessen the chance of prolapse.

Stress Reduction: Stress may dramatically impair pelvic floor health, leading to muscular tension and dysfunction. Yoga's focus on deep breathing, relaxation, and mindfulness may help you manage stress, decrease muscular tension, and increase general well-being.

Improved Body Image: Pelvic floor dysfunction may adversely affect a woman's body image and self-esteem. Yoga encourages body acceptance and self-love, helping you create a healthy connection with your body and embrace your feminine power.

In essence, yoga offers a tremendous arsenal for women trying to regain their pelvic health and vitality.

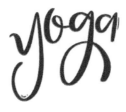

Who Can Benefit: From New Moms to Menopause and Beyond

Pelvic floor yoga is good for women of all ages and stages of life:

New Moms: Pregnancy and delivery may dramatically alter the pelvic floor, leading to weakening, incontinence, or prolapse. Yoga may help restore strength and function, facilitating speedier recovery and decreasing long-term consequences.

Women Experiencing Menopause: Hormonal changes during menopause might lead to pelvic floor weakness and dryness. Yoga may assist in maintaining muscular tone, enhance circulation, and minimize soreness.

Women with Pelvic discomfort: Yoga's gentle stretches and relaxation practices may help decrease pelvic discomfort associated with illnesses like endometriosis, interstitial cystitis, or vulvodynia.

Athletes: High-impact exercises may put stress on the pelvic floor. Yoga may help athletes develop and preserve these muscles, reducing injuries and boosting performance.

Any Woman Seeking to Enhance Pelvic Health: Even if you don't have any particular pelvic floor difficulties, yoga may be a proactive strategy to maintain pelvic health, develop core strength, and promote general well-being.

Chapter 2: Core Connection

Building a strong foundation starts from the inside out. As you engage your core in these exercises, you're laying the groundwork for improved stability, better posture, and enhanced pelvic floor function. Every small effort you put into connecting with your core brings you closer to a stronger, more resilient body. Stay committed, and let each movement remind you of your inner strength

The Core: Your Body's Power Center

Your core is more than just your six-pack abs; it's a complex system of muscles that goes well beyond your superficial abdominal muscles. It contains your deep abdominal muscles (transverse abdominis), pelvic floor muscles, diaphragm, and multifidus (deep back muscles). Together, these muscles create a supporting corset around your trunk, giving stability, balance, and power to your whole body.

The Role of the Core in Pelvic Health

A strong and functioning core is vital for pelvic health. Your deep abdominal muscles, in particular, serve a key function in supporting your pelvic organs and sustaining continence. They act in cooperation with your pelvic floor muscles to provide intra-abdominal pressure, which helps avoid leaks and prolapse.

When your core is weak or uneven, it may place unnecessary stress on your pelvic floor, leading to dysfunction and a variety of pelvic health concerns. That's why exercising your deep abdominal muscles is a major component of pelvic floor yoga.

Exercise 1

Finding Your Deep Core Muscles

Unlike your superficial abdominal muscles, which are easier to see and feel, your deep core muscles are more subtle and take a little more effort to activate. Here's a simple exercise to help you connect with your transverse abdominis:

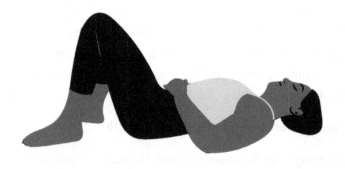

1. Lie on your back with your knees bent and your feet resting flat on the floor.
2. Place your fingers on your lower abdomen, right inside your hip bones.

3. Take a deep breath in, allowing your tummy to expand.
4. As you exhale, gently bring your navel towards your spine, experiencing a tiny tightness beneath your fingers.
5. Hold this moderate contraction for a few seconds, breathing normally.
6. Release and repeat.

For many women, the pelvic floor remains a mysterious and elusive part of their anatomy. It's not something we can readily see or touch, making it challenging to connect with and understand. However, raising awareness of these muscles is the first step in enhancing both their general health and function in the pelvis.

While the pelvic floor may seem elusive, several techniques can help you pinpoint its location and establish a connection with these essential muscles. Each method offers a slightly different perspective, allowing you to explore and understand your pelvic floor from various angles.

Exercise 2

The "Stop-and-Start" Method

How it works: This technique leverages a familiar function of the pelvic floor—controlling the flow of urine.

Steps:

1. While urinating, try to gently stop the flow midstream.
2. Notice the muscles you engage to do this—that's your pelvic floor!
3. Release the muscles and allow the flow to resume.

Important Note: This method is helpful for initial identification, but avoid using it frequently as it can disrupt healthy bladder habits.

Exercise 3

The "Kegel Squeeze"

How it works: Kegel exercises directly target the pelvic floor muscles, helping you isolate and feel them contract.

Steps:

1. Consider that you are attempting to prevent yourself from urinating or passing gas.
2. Squeeze and lift the muscles around your urethra, vagina (if applicable), and anus.
3. Hold the contraction, after a few seconds of holding the contraction, release it.

4. Repeat several times.

Exercise 4

The "Visualization Technique"

How it works: This method relies on mental imagery to connect with your pelvic floor.

Steps:

1. Find a comfortable seated position.
2. Take several deep breaths while closing your eyes.
3. Visualize the base of your pelvis as a hammock or a bowl.
4. Imagine the muscles raising and supporting your pelvic organs.
5. Gently contract and release these visualized muscles.

Exercise 5

The "Prop Assist"

How it works: Utilizing props can provide tactile feedback, making it easier to feel the pelvic floor engage.

Steps:

1. Lie down on your back, bending your knees and placing your feet flat on the ground.
2. Place a small ball or yoga block between your thighs.

3. Gently squeeze the prop as you contract your pelvic floor muscles.
4. You should feel the muscles lift and tighten around the prop.

Exercise 6

The "Mindful Breathing Connection"

How it works: This approach links the natural movement of your diaphragm during breathing to your pelvic floor.

Steps:

1. Lie on your back with knees bent.
2. Inhale deeply, allowing your belly to rise and your pelvic floor to relax and expand.
3. Breathe out slowly, gently activating and lifting your pelvic floor while pulling your belly inward.

Engaging Your Core in Yoga Poses

Once you've discovered your deep core muscles, you can start integrating them into your yoga practice. Here are some tips:

Engage your core as you exhale, pulling your navel towards your spine. This helps balance your pelvis and protect your lower back.

Avoid arching your back or tucking your tailbone. Aim for a natural curvature in your lower back.

Begin with easy positions that enable you to concentrate on core activation without sacrificing form As you build strength and awareness, you can progress to more challenging poses. Props like blocks or blankets may help you maintain good alignment and reduce strain. If you experience any pain or discomfort, back off or change the stance.

Yoga Poses for Core Strength

Exercise 7

Plank Pose (Phalakasana)

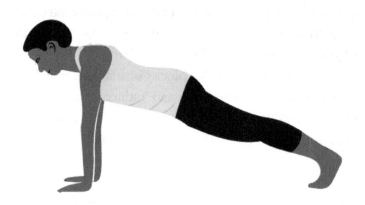

Steps:

1. Begin on your hands and knees, aligning your wrists directly under your shoulders and your knees beneath your hips.
2. Step your feet back one at a time, going into a high push-up posture.
3. Make sure your body forms a straight line from your head to your heels, engaging your core and glutes.
4. Press your hands onto the mat, stretch your fingers wide, and look slightly ahead.

5. Hold the position for many breaths, keeping a steady and regulated breath.

Beginners' Tips:

- If holding a complete plank is tough, start with a reduced plank on your forearms.
- Keep your core engaged to minimize drooping in the lower back.
- If you feel any tension in your wrists, consider utilizing yoga blocks beneath your hands.

Benefits:

- Strengthens the whole core, including the deep abdominal muscles and pelvic floor.
- Improves posture and stability.
- Builds upper body and arm strength.

Watch out for:

- **Sagging in the lower back:** Keep your core engaged and prevent arching your back.
- **Shoulder tension:** Keep your shoulders away from your ears and push your hands into the mat
- **Wrist trouble:** If you have wrist pain, adjust the position by practicing on your forearms or using yoga blocks.

Variations:

1. **Forearm Plank:** Rest on your forearms instead of your hands, keeping your elbows aligned beneath your shoulders.
2. **Side Plank:** Balance on one hand and the outside edge of the same foot, stacking your feet or staggering them for extra stability.
3. **Plank with Leg Lift:** Lift one leg at a time while keeping a solid plank posture.

Exercise 8

Bird Dog (Parsva Balasana)

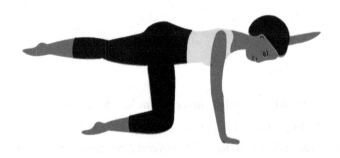

Steps:

1. Start on your hands and knees with your wrists aligned under your shoulders and your knees beneath your hips.

2. Reach your right arm forward while extending your left leg back, keeping your hips level and your core engaged.
3. Reach through your fingers and heel, keeping a long spine.
4. Hold the position for a few breaths, then switch sides by extending your left arm and right leg.

Beginners' Tips:

- If the balance is tough, keep your sight down towards the floor.
- Focus on maintaining your hips level and core engaged to prevent twisting or arching your back.
- If you encounter any pain in your lower back, alter your posture by maintaining your knee on the ground or practicing it against a wall for support.

Benefits:

- Improves core stability and coordination.
- Strengthens the back and abdominal muscles.
- Enhances balance and pelvic floor involvement.

Watch out for:

- **Arching or rounding the back:** Keep your spine neutral throughout the position.
- **Twisting in the hips:** Keep your hips level and face the ground.
- **Strain in the neck:** Keep your neck neutral and glance down towards the floor.

Variations:

1. **Bird Dog with Knee Tap:** Instead of extending your leg completely, tap your knee to the ground and pull it back up.
2. **Bird Dog with Arm and Leg Circles:** Once you've gained stability, try forming little circles with your extended arm and leg.

Exercise 9

Bridge Pose (Setu Bandhasana)

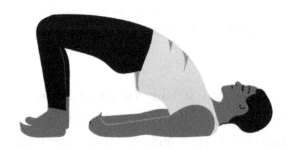

Steps:

1. Lie on your back with your knees bent and your feet flat on the floor, spaced hip-width apart.
2. Press your feet and arms into the ground as you raise your hips off the mat.

3. To raise your hips higher, place your fingers behind your pelvis and extend your arms downward.
4. Keep your thighs and inner feet parallel.
5. Hold for several breaths, then release by gently lowering your hips back to the mat.

Beginners' Tips

- If you feel any tension in your neck, maintain it neutral or lay a blanket beneath your shoulders for support.
- Avoid raising your hips too high; concentrate on maintaining a comfortable lift.
- If your feet turn out, insert a block between your thighs to assist in maintaining them parallel.

Benefits:

- Strengthens the glutes, hamstrings, and deep core muscles.
- Stretches the chest, shoulders, and hip flexors.
- Improves spinal flexibility.
- Can help reduce menstruation cramps and exhaustion.

Watch out for:

- **Neck strain:** Keep your neck neutral and avoid staring up towards the ceiling.
- **Overhanging the back:** Focus on elevating your hips without overhanging your lower back.

- **Knee discomfort:** If you feel knee pain, tuck a rolled-up blanket beneath your knees for support.

Variations:

1. **Bridge Pose with Block:** Place a yoga block beneath your sacrum for a more supported and restful alternative.
2. **Single-Leg Bridge:** Lift one leg towards the ceiling while keeping a bridge stance with the other leg.

Exercise 10

Boat Pose (Navasana)

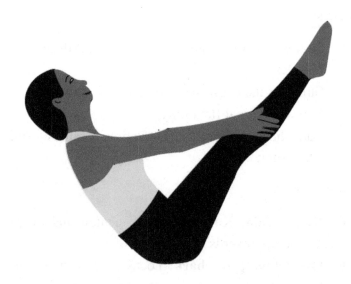

Steps:

1. With your feet flat and knees bent, take a seat on the floor.
2. With your shin parallel to the floor, incline your back slightly and lift your feet off the ground.
3. Maintain your balance on your sitting bones by using your core.
4. Arms extended forward, parallel to the ground, palms facing one another.
5. For a more advanced variant, straighten your legs, producing a V-shape with your torso.

Beginners' Tips:

- If balance is tough, keep your hands behind your thighs for support.
- Maintaining a straight back and an engaged core is important.
- Start by holding the position for a few breaths and progressively extend the length as you grow stronger.

Benefits:

- Strengthens the core muscles, especially the deep abdominals and pelvic floor.
- Improves balance and coordination.
- Stimulates the organs of the abdomen.

Watch out for:

- **Rounding your back:** To reduce tension, keep your back straight.

- **Overextending your neck:** Keep your neck neutral and glance ahead.
- If you have any neck, back, or shoulder issues, visit a yoga teacher before trying this posture.

Variations:

1. **Half Boat Pose:** Rather of straightening your legs, maintain a shin-to-floor position.
2. **Boat Pose with a block:** To help engage your inner thighs, hold a block between your thighs.

Exercise 11

Chair Pose (Utkatasana)

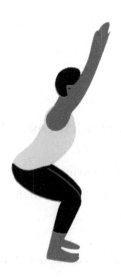

Steps:

1. Stand with your feet hip-width apart.
2. Bend your knees and drop your hips as if you're sitting on a chair.
3. Keep your back straight and your core tight.
4. Raise your arms upward, palms facing each other.

Beginners' Tips:

- If your heels rise off the ground, tuck a rolled-up blanket beneath them for support.
- Keep your weight on your heels and avoid leaning forward too far.
- If you encounter any knee discomfort, alter the position by not bending your knees as deeply.

Benefits:

- Strengthens the legs, glutes, and core muscles, especially the pelvic floor.
- Improves balance and posture.
- Stretches the shoulders and chest.

Watch out for:

- **Knee pain:** Avoid bending your knees beyond a comfortable range.
- **Rounding your back:** Maintain a straight back and a contracted core.
- If you have any knee or ankle issues, see a yoga teacher before trying this position.

Variations:

Chair Pose with a block: Activate your inner thighs with the help of a block held between your thighs.

Chair Pose with a twist: Twist your body to one side, hooking your elbow outside the opposing knee.

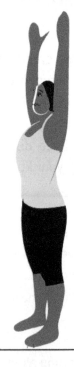

Mountain Pose (Tadasana). Take note of this POSE

Exercise 12

Warrior III (Virabhadrasana III)

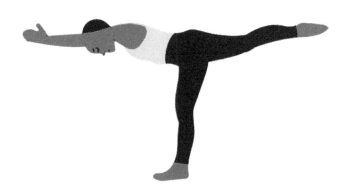

Steps:

1. Start in Mountain Pose (Tadasana).
2. Step your right foot back and raise your left leg parallel to the floor.
3. As you maintain your back straight and your core active, bend forward at the hips.
4. Extend your arms, keeping your palms facing one another.

Beginners' Tips:

- If balance is problematic, use a wall or chair for support.
- Keep your focus on a fixed spot in front of you to assist in maintaining balance.
- Focus on using your core and pelvic floor muscles for stability.

Benefits:

- Improves balance and coordination.
- Strengthens the legs, glutes, and core muscles, especially the pelvic floor.
- Stretches the hamstrings and calves.

Watch out for:

1. Arching your back: Maintain a straight back to minimize tension.
2. Dropping your elevated leg: Keep your lifted leg parallel to the floor.
3. If you have any back, hip, or ankle issues, visit a yoga teacher before trying this posture.

Variations:

1. **Warrior III with a block:** Place a block beneath your front foot for support.
2. **Warrior III with hands on hips**: If balance is problematic, lay your hands on your hips.

Exercise 13

Goddess Pose (Utkata Konasana)

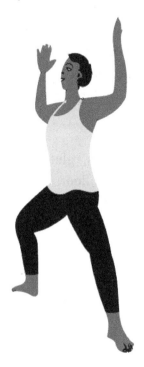

Steps:

1. Place your feet wider than hip-width apart and gently turn your toes out as you stand.
2. Bend your knees and drop your hips until your thighs are parallel to the floor.
3. Maintain a straight back and a contracted core.
4. Raise your arms out to the sides, palms facing each other.

Beginners' Tips:

- If your heels rise off the ground, tuck a rolled-up blanket beneath them for support.
- Keep your knees aligned with your toes and avoid letting them fall inward.
- If you encounter any knee discomfort, alter the position by not bending your knees as deeply.

Benefits:

- Strengthens the legs, glutes, and core muscles, especially the pelvic floor.
- Opens the hips and groin.
- Improves circulation and energy flow.

Watch out for:

- **Knee pain:** Avoid bending your knees beyond a comfortable range.
- **Rounding your back:** Maintain a straight back and a tight core.

Variations:

1. **Goddess Pose with a block:** Activate your inner thighs with the help of a block held between your thighs.
2. **Goddess Pose with arm variations:** You may lift your arms aloft or bring your hands together in front of your chest.

Chapter 3: Gentle Flows: Warming Up and Connecting with Your Body

Warming up isn't just about preparing your muscles—it's about connecting with your body and setting the tone for your practice. These gentle flows invite you to listen to your body, awaken your senses, and create a harmonious relationship with your movements. Embrace this time as a moment to honor your body's needs, and let it guide you toward a more mindful practice.

These easy routines are meant to prepare your body for deeper pelvic floor yoga practice by boosting circulation, enhancing mobility, and fostering body awareness. Remember to focus on your breath and move carefully during each flow.

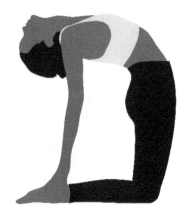

Yoga Pose

Exercise 14

Cat-Cow (Marjaryasana-Bitilasana)

Steps:

1. Start on your hands and knees, positioning your wrists under your shoulders and knees under your hips (tabletop posture).
2. Inhale, arch your back, sink your tummy towards the mat, elevate your tailbone, and gaze upwards **(Cow Pose).**
3. Exhale, curve your spine towards the ceiling, tuck your tailbone, and drag your pubic bone forward **(Cat Pose).**
4. Continue flowing between these two positions, connecting your movement with your breath.

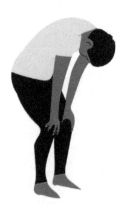 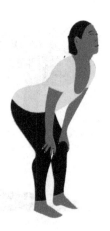

Beginners' Tips:

- As you spread your hands shoulder-width apart, so do the same with your knees.
- Move slowly and deliberately, concentrating on the link between your breath and movement.
- If you encounter any wrist ache, you can interlace your fingers and push your knuckles into the mat.

Benefits:

- Improves spinal flexibility and mobility.
- Massages the abdominal organs, improving digestion.
- Increases blood flow to the spine and pelvic region.
- Enhances pelvic floor awareness and harmony with the breath.
- Reduces stress and tension.

Watch out for:

- Overarching your back in Cow Pose: Keep a small bend in your elbows and engage your core to cushion your lower back.
- Collapsing in your shoulders in Cat Pose: Keep your shoulders away from your ears and press your hands into the mat.
- If you encounter any neck strain, keep your eyes neutral instead of gazing up in Cow Pose.

Variations:

1. **Seated Cat-Cow:** Perform the same action while seated on a chair, rounding and arching your spine with your breath.
2. **Cat-Cow with pelvic floor focus:** As you exhale into Cat Pose, softly engage and elevate your pelvic floor muscles. As you inhale into Cow Pose, relax your pelvic floor.
3.

Exercise 15

Pelvic Tilts

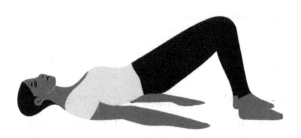

Steps:

1. Lay flat on your back with your feet flat on the ground and your legs bent.

2. Inhale, softly arch your lower back, pressing your navel towards the floor.
3. Exhale, tilt your pelvis back, pressing your lower back into the mat and bringing your pubic bone towards your navel.
4. Maintain the back-and-forth tilt of your pelvis in time with your breathing.

Beginners' Tips:

- Keep your motions modest and controlled.
- Focus on isolating the action to your pelvis and lower back.
- You can place your hands on your lower abdomen to feel the slight motions of your pelvic floor.

Benefits:

- Enhances pelvic mobility and flexibility.
- Strengthens the deep core muscles, especially the transverse abdominis.
- Improves awareness of the pelvic floor muscles.
- Can help reduce lower back pain.

Watch out for:

- **Overarching your back:** Keep the action modest and controlled, avoiding any tension.
- **Engaging your glutes or hamstrings:** Focus on isolating the movement to your pelvis.

Variations:

1. **Seated pelvic tilts:** Perform the same exercise while seated on a chair, keeping your feet flat on the floor.
2. **Pelvic tilts with Kegels:** As you tilt your pelvis back, gently activate your pelvic floor muscles.

Exercise 16

Child's Pose to Downward-Facing Dog (Balasana to Adho Mukha Svanasana)

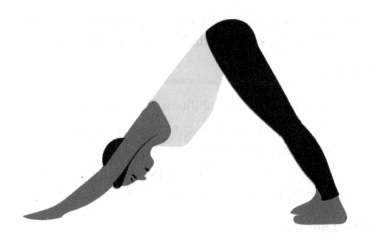

Steps:

1. Start on your hands and knees in a tabletop posture.
2. Breath out, pull your hips back to your heels, and lay your forehead on the mat (Child's Pose).

3. Inhale, raise your hips up and back, straightening your legs and generating an inverted V-shape with your body (Downward-Facing Dog).
4. Keep your hands shoulder-width apart, feet hip-width apart, and heels extending towards the floor.
5. Hold for several breaths, then exhale back into Child's Pose.
6. Make many repetitions of the flow, synchronizing your movements with your breathing.

Beginners' Tips:

- If your hamstrings feel tight, retain a tiny bend in your knees.
- Focus on stretching your spine and reaching your sit bones towards the ceiling in Downward-Facing Dog.
- If you encounter any wrist ache, you can interlace your fingers and push your knuckles into the mat.

Benefits:

- Gently stretch the spine, hamstrings, and calves.
- Enhances the blood supply to the brain and circulation.
- Calms the mind and relieves stress.
- Encourages deep breathing and relaxation.

Watch out for:

- **Rounding your back in Downward-Facing Dog:** Keep your core engaged and push your chest towards your thighs.
- **Hyperextending your knees:** Keep a modest bend in your knees if your hamstrings feel tight.
- If you have any wrist, shoulder, or back issues, visit a yoga instructor before attempting this sequence.

Variations:

1. **Child's Pose with a bolster:** Place a bolster under your torso for added support.
2. **Downward-Facing Dog with a Block:** Place a block beneath your heels if they don't reach the floor.
3. **Puppy Pose:** From tabletop posture, move your hands forward while maintaining your hips above your knees, allowing your chest to melt toward the floor.

Exercise 17

Standing Forward Fold to Halfway Lift (Uttanasana to Ardha Uttanasana)

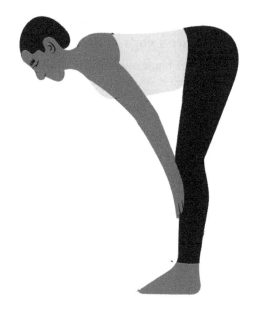

Steps:

1. Stand with your feet hip-width apart.
2. Breathe out, fold forward from your hips, reaching towards your toes or shins (Uttanasana).
3. Inhale, elevate your torso halfway, maintaining your back flat and core engaged (Ardha Uttanasana).

4. Gaze forward, stretching your spine.
5. Exhale, fold back down into Uttanasana.
6. Make many repetitions of the flow, synchronizing your movements with your breathing.

Beginners' Tips:

- If you can't reach your toes, bend your knees slightly or place a yoga strap around your feet.
- Maintain a flat back and refrain from arching your spine.
- Focus on stretching your spine with each breath.

Benefits:

- Stretches the hamstrings, calves, and spine.
- Enhances the blood supply to the brain and circulation.
- Calms the mind and relieves stress.
- Gently stimulates the core muscles.

Watch out for:

- **Rounding your back:** Keep your back flat, even if it means bending your knees.
- **Hyperextending your knees:** Keep a modest bend in your knees if your hamstrings feel tight.
- If you have any back or hamstring issues, visit a yoga instructor before doing this sequence.

Variations:

1. **Wide-Legged Forward Fold:** Step your feet widely apart and fold forward, allowing your body to dangle between your legs.
2. **Halfway Lift with blocks:** Place blocks beneath your hands for assistance if you can't reach the floor.

Exercise 18

Mountain Pose with Arm Circles (Tadasana with arm circles):

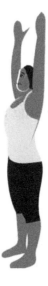

Steps:

1. Stand tall with your feet hip-width apart, toes looking front.

2. Ground your feet into the mat and stretch your spine, reaching the crown of your head towards the ceiling.
3. Let your shoulders relax, allowing your arms to rest naturally by your sides.
4. As you inhale, stretch your arms out to the sides and reach them overhead, with your palms facing each other.
5. On the exhale, bring your arms back down to your sides.
6. Keep circling your arms, synchronizing the movement with your breath.

Beginners' Tips:

- Maintain core engagement and avoid straining your lower back.
- Relax your shoulders and neck.
- Concentrate on maintaining a steady, even breath throughout the exercise.

Benefits:

- Improves posture and body awareness.
- Warms up the shoulders and upper back.
- Increases circulation and energy flow.
- Promotes deep breathing and relaxation.

Watch out for:

- **Overarching your lower back:** Engage your core and maintain your pelvis neutral.

- **Tensing your shoulders:** Relax your shoulders and maintain your neck long.

Variations:

1. **Reverse arm circles:** Circle your arms in the other way.
2. **Arm circles with varied hand positions:** Experiment with palms facing up, down, or forward.

Exercise 19

Seated Spinal Twist (Parivrtta Sukhasana)

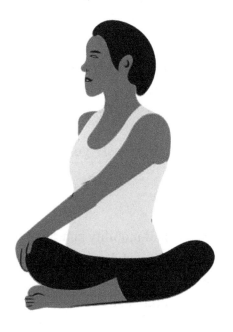

Steps:

1. Cross your legs and sit comfortably on the floor in the Sukhasana or Easy Pose.
2. Grind your sit bones into the mat while elongating your spine.
3. Taking a breath, raise your right arm toward the ceiling.
4. Exhale, rotate your torso to the left, resting your right hand on the floor behind you and your left hand on your right knee.
5. Gaze over your left shoulder, keeping your neck long and relaxed.
6. Breathe in for a few breaths, then exhale and repeat on the other side.

Beginners' Tips:

- If your hips are stiff, sit on a block or blanket to raise your seat.
- Do not round your back; instead, maintain a long spine.
- Don't push the twist; go only as far as feels comfortable.

Benefits:

- Increases spinal mobility and flexibility.
- Massages the abdominal organs, improving digestion.
- Improves posture and decreases stress.

Watch out for:

1. Rounding your back: Keep your spine long and prevent collapsing in your chest.
2. Straining your neck: Remain neutral with your neck and refrain from over-twisting.

Variations:

1. **Seated twist using a strap:** If you can't reach your back foot, use a strap to aid the twist.
2. **Revolved Chair Pose:** Perform a sitting twist while in Chair Pose for a more strenuous variant.

Exercise 20

Supine Spinal Twist (Supta Matsyendrasana)

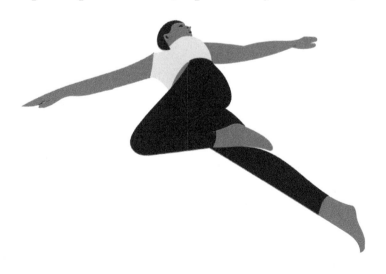

Steps:

1. Lay yourself on your back, legs bent, and feet flat on the floor.
2. Make a T-shape with your arms extended outward.
3. Exhale, lower your knees to the right, keeping your shoulders on the mat.
4. Turn your head to the left, glancing over your left shoulder.
5. Breathe in for a few breaths, then exhale and repeat on the opposite side.

Beginners' Tips:

- If your knees don't comfortably reach the floor, lay a block or blanket under them for support.
- Keep your shoulders relaxed and push against the mat.
- If you feel any tension in your neck, keep your head facing the ceiling.

Benefits:

- Gently stretch the spine, hips, and shoulders.
- Massages the abdominal organs, improving digestion.
- Enhances circulation and lymphatic flow.
- Reduces stress and tension.

Watch out for:

- **Forcing the twist:** Go only as far as feels comfortable, avoiding any discomfort or strain.
- **Lifting your shoulders off the mat:** Keep your shoulders loose and planted.
- If you have any back, neck, or shoulder issues, visit a yoga instructor before attempting this posture.

Variations:

1. **The supine twist with a strap:** If your knees don't reach the floor, use a strap to gently assist them down.
2. **The supine twist with eagle legs:** Cross your right thigh over your left and wrap your right foot around your left calf for a deeper hip stretch.

Exercise 21

Legs-up-the-Wall Pose (Viparita Karani)

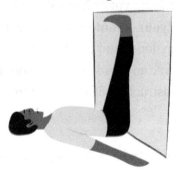

Steps:

1. Sit sideways against a wall, with your hip near to the wall.
2. Gently swing your legs up the wall while you lie back on the floor.
3. Let your arms rest by your sides, with your palms facing upward.
4. Close your eyes and allow your entire body to relax.
5. Hold for 5-10 minutes, breathing deeply and evenly.

Beginners' Tips:

- If your hamstrings feel tight, step slightly away from the wall or lay a blanket under your hips for support.
- If you notice any soreness in your lower back, lay a little rolled-up cloth beneath your sacrum.

- You may also practice this posture with your legs resting on a chair instead of the wall.

Benefits:

- Promotes relaxation and relieves weariness.
- Improves circulation and lymphatic drainage.
- Relieves swelling ankles and feet.
- Calms the mind and relieves stress.

Watch out for:

- **Neck strain:** If your neck feels strained, tuck a blanket or pillow under your head for support.
- **Discomfort in the lower back:** If you suffer any discomfort, modify your position or lay a cloth beneath your sacrum.
- If you have any glaucoma or high blood pressure, see a healthcare practitioner before attempting this position.

Variations:

1. **Legs-up-the-wall using a strap:** position a strap around your thighs to assist in maintaining your legs in position.
2. **Legs-up-the-wall with a bolster:** Place a bolster under your hips for more support and comfort.
3. **Waterfall pose:** From the Legs-up-the-Wall Pose, slowly extend your legs wide apart, allowing them to fall towards the sides like a waterfall.

Chapter 4: Strengthening Poses: Building Pelvic Floor Power

Strength comes from consistent, mindful effort. As you work through these strengthening poses, imagine the power you're cultivating in your pelvic floor muscles. This is your journey toward greater stability and support, not just in your yoga practice but in everyday life. With each pose, you're investing in a future where you feel stronger and more empowered.

Exercise 22

Warrior II (Virabhadrasana II)

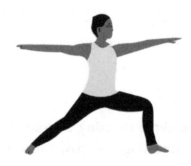

Steps:

1. Start in Mountain Pose (Tadasana).
2. Step your right foot back about 4 feet, turning it 90 degrees to the right.

3. Position your left heel in line with the arch of your right foot.
4. Bend your left knee until it is squarely over your left ankle, maintaining your right leg straight.
5. Stretch your arms out to the sides, parallel to the floor, with your palms facing downward.
6. Gaze ahead over your left hand.
7. Hold for several breaths, then exchange sides.

Beginners' Tips:

- Keep your front knee bent at a 90-degree angle, tracking over your ankle.
- Activate your core and keep your back straight.
- If you feel any tension in your knees, expand your stance or place a block under your front heel.

Benefits:

- Strengthens the legs, ankles, and core.
- Improves balance and stability.
- Stretches the hips, groin, and chest.
- Increases stamina and attention.

Watch out for:

- **Front knee sinking inward:** Maintain alignment of your front knee with your ankle.
- **Back heel lifting off the ground:** Press your back heel down into the mat.
- **Neck strain:** Keep your neck neutral and glance forward.

Variations:

1. **Warrior II with a block:** Place a block under your front hand for assistance if you can't reach the floor.
2. **Reverse Warrior:** From Warrior II, reach your front arm up towards the ceiling and your rear arm down towards your back leg.

Exercise 23

Triangle Pose (Trikonasana)

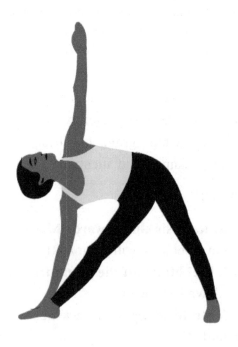

Steps:

1. Start in Mountain Pose (Tadasana).
2. Step your feet wide apart, roughly 3-4 feet.
3. Rotate your right foot outward 90 degrees and turn your left foot in slightly.
4. Stretch your arms out to the sides, keeping them parallel to the floor.
5. Inhale, stretch your spine and exhale, reach your right hand towards your ankle or shin (or a block).
6. Extend your left arm towards the ceiling, keeping your palm facing down.
7. Gaze up towards your left hand.
8. Hold for several breaths, then exchange sides.

Beginners' Tips:

- Maintain a straight back and avoid arching your spine
- Don't worry about reaching your ankle; focus on stretching your spine and maintaining your chest wide.
- Use a block beneath your hand for support if needed.

Benefits:

- Stretches and strengthens the legs, ankles, and core.
- Improves balance and stability.
- Opens the chest and shoulders.

- Promotes pelvic floor awareness and involvement.

Watch out for:

- **Hyperextending your front knee:** Keep a modest bend in your front knee.
- **Collapsing in your chest:** Keep your chest open and your front arm stretching towards the ceiling.
- **Neck strain:** If your neck feels strained, maintain your gaze forward instead of gazing up.

Variations:

1. **Triangle Pose with a block:** Place a block under your hand for support.
2. **Revolved Triangle Pose:** From Triangle Pose, twist your torso and extend your front arm underneath your front leg.

Exercise 24

Extended Side Angle Pose (Parsvottanasana)

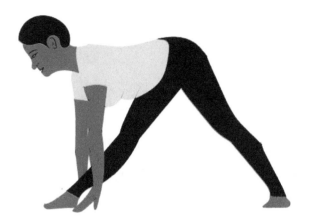

Steps:

1. Start in Mountain Pose (Tadasana).
2. Step your right foot back about three to four feet, turning it slightly outward.
3. Keep your left foot looking forward.
4. Fold forward from your hips, maintaining your back straight.
5. Position your hands on the floor or on blocks beside your front foot.
6. Gaze forward or down towards the floor.
7. Hold for several breaths, then exchange sides.

Beginners' Tips:

- Bend your front knee slightly if your hamstrings feel tight.
- Maintain a straight back and avoid arching your spine
- Use bricks beneath your hands for support if needed.

Benefits:

- Strengthens the legs, ankles, and core.
- Stretches the hamstrings, calves, and spine.
- Improves balance and stability.
- Promotes pelvic floor engagement.

Watch out for:

- **Rounding your back:** Keep your back straight, even if it means bending your front knee.
- **Hyperextending your front knee:** Keep a modest bend in your front knee.
- **Neck strain:** If your neck feels strained, keep your look down towards the floor.

Variations:

1. **Extended Side Angle Pose with a chair:** Place your hands on a chair for support.
2. **Revolved Extended Side Angle Pose:** From Extended Side Angle Pose, twist your torso and reach your front arm towards the ceiling.

Exercise 25

High Lunge (Anjaneyasana)

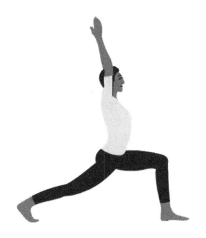

Steps:

1. Start in Mountain Pose (Tadasana).
2. Step your right foot back approximately 3-4 feet.
3. Bend your left knee till it is squarely over your left ankle.
4. Keep your right leg straight and your back heel raised.
5. Raise your arms upward, palms facing each other.

Beginners' Tips:

- Ensure your front knee stays aligned with your ankle.
- Activate your core and keep your back straight.

- If you feel any strain in your knees, shorten your stance or throw a blanket under your back knee.

Benefits:

- Strengthens the legs, glutes, and core.
- Stretches the hip flexors and quads.
- Improves balance and stability.
- Promotes pelvic floor awareness.

Watch out for:

- **Front knee sinking inward:** Ensure your front knee is aligned with your ankle.
- **Back heel lifting off the ground:** Press your back heel down towards the mat.
- **Arching your back:** Keep your core activated and your back straight.

Variations:

1. High Lunge using a block: Place a block under your front hand for support.
2. Crescent Lunge: From High Lunge, bend your back knee and reach your back arm towards the ceiling.

Exercise 26

Tree Pose (Vrksasana)

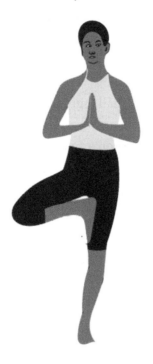

Steps:

1. Start in Mountain Pose (Tadasana) with your feet positioned hip-width apart.
2. Shift your weight onto your left foot and bend your right knee, bringing the sole of your right foot to your inner left thigh, calf, or ankle. Make sure it's not directly on your knee joint.
3. Press your foot and leg together, gaining stability.

4. Bring your hands to your chest in prayer position (Anjali Mudra) or extend them overhead.
5. Hold for several breaths, focusing on your balance and pelvic floor engagement.
6. Repeat on the other side.

Beginners' Tips:

- If balancing is challenging, use a wall or chair for support.
- Focus your focus on a fixed place in front of you to help maintain balance.
- If you can't bring your foot to your inner thigh, place it on your calf or ankle.

Benefits:

- Improves balance, coordination, and focus.
- Strengthens the legs, ankles, and core, especially the pelvic floor.
- Stretches the hips, groin, and inner thighs.
- Promotes grounding and stability.

Watch out for:

- **Hyperextending your standing knee:** Keep a modest bend in your standing knee.
- **Placing your foot on your knee joint:** This might generate tension on the knee.
- **Losing your balance:** If you start to wobble, softly lower your foot and try again.

Variations:

1. **Tree Pose with Eyes Closed:** Once you feel stable, consider closing your eyes to deepen the balance challenge.

2. **Tree Pose with arm variations:** Experiment with different arm positions, such as stretching your arms overhead or interlacing your fingers behind your back.

Exercise 27

Bridge Pose with Block (Sctu Bandhasana with block)

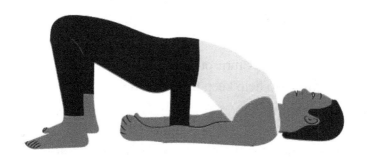

Steps:

1. Lie on your back with your legs bent and feet flat on the floor, hip-width apart.
2. Place a yoga block under your sacrum, adjusting the height as needed for comfort.
3. Press your feet and arms into the ground as you lift your hips off the mat.
4. Interlace your fingers under your pelvis and press your arms down to elevate your hips a bit higher.
5. Keep your thighs and inner feet parallel.
6. Hold for several breaths, then release by gently lowering your hips back to the mat.

Beginners' Tips:

- Start with the lowest height on the block and progressively increase as you feel comfortable.
- If you feel any strain in your neck, maintain it neutral or lay a blanket beneath your shoulders for support.
- If your feet turn out, insert a block between your thighs to help keep them parallel.

Benefits:

- Strengthens the glutes, hamstrings, and deep core muscles, including the pelvic floor.
- Stretches the chest, shoulders, and hip flexors.
- Improves spinal flexibility.

- Can help reduce menstruation cramps and exhaustion.
- The block intensifies the pelvic floor engagement.

Watch out for:

- **Neck strain:** Keep your neck neutral and avoid staring up towards the ceiling.
- **Overarching the back:** Concentrate on lifting your hips while avoiding an overarch in your lower back
- **Knee pain:** If you feel knee pain, tuck a rolled-up blanket under your knees for support.

Variations:

1. Bridge Pose without a block: Practice the standard Bridge Pose without the block for a less strenuous stretch.
2. Single-Leg Bridge with block: Lift one leg towards the ceiling while keeping a bridge stance with the other leg and the block under your sacrum.

Exercise 28

Reclining Bound Angle Pose (Supta Baddha Konasana)

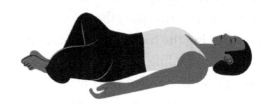

Steps:

1. Recline on your back with your legs bent and your feet flat on the floor.
2. Bring the soles of your feet together and allow your knees to fall open to the sides.
3. Place blocks or blankets under your knees for support if needed.
4. Let your arms rest by your sides with your palms facing up.
5. Close your eyes and relax your whole body
6. Hold for several minutes, breathing deeply and evenly.

Beginners' Tips:

- Use props for support: Place blocks or blankets under your knees to alleviate any tightness in your hips and groin.
- Focus on your breath: Breathe deeply into your abdomen and allow your body to relax with each exhale.

Benefits:

- Gently extend the inner thighs, groin, and hips.
- Promotes relaxation and release of tension in the pelvic floor muscles.
- Improves circulation to the pelvic area.
- Can help alleviate period cramps and discomfort.

Watch out for:

- **Knee pain:** If you suffer any knee pain, modify the props or come out of the pose.
- **Overstretching:** Avoid pulling your knees open; let gravity do the work.

Variations:

1. **Supta Baddha Konasana with a bolster:** Place a bolster under your spine for a more supported and restorative variant.
2. **Supta Baddha Konasana with an eye cushion:** Add an eye pillow to increase relaxation and deepen the pose.

Exercise 29

Squat Pose (Malasana)

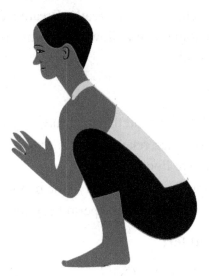

Steps:

1. Stand with your feet somewhat wider than hip-width apart, toes turned out slightly.
2. Bend your knees and lower your hips down towards the floor, aiming to bring your thighs parallel to the ground.
3. Bring your palms together in front of your chest and use your elbows to gently push your knees open.
4. Maintain a straight back and engage your core.
5. Hold for several breaths, then slowly climb back up to standing.

Beginners' Tips:

- If your heels rise off the ground, tuck a rolled-up blanket under them for support.
- If maintaining balance is challenging, practice with your back against a wall.
- If your hips are tight, position a block under your sitting bones for support.

Benefits:

- Strengthens the legs, glutes, and core muscles, especially the pelvic floor.
- Stretches the ankles, groin, and hips.
- Improves digestion and excretion.
- Promotes pelvic floor awareness and relaxation.

Watch out for:

- **Knee pain:** Avoid bending your knees beyond a comfortable range.
- **Rounding your back:** Maintain a straight back and engage your core.
- If you have any knee, ankle, or hip issues, visit a yoga instructor before attempting this posture.

Variations

1. **Garland Pose (Malasana) using a block:** Place a brick under your sitting bones for support.
2. **Garland Pose with a strap:** If you can't pull your palms together, hold a strap between your hands.

Chapter 5

Lengthening Poses: Releasing Tension and Improving Flexibility

Flexibility is a form of freedom—freedom from tension, stiffness, and restriction. In these lengthening poses, allow yourself to release what no longer serves you. Each stretch is an opportunity to let go, create space, and invite ease into your body. Recall, flexibility comes with patience and persistence, so treat yourself with kindness as you expand your range of motion.

Exercise 29

Pigeon Pose (Eka Pada Rajakapotasana)

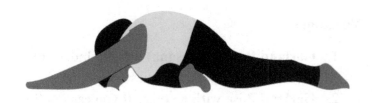

Steps:

1. Begin in a tabletop position, with your hands and knees on the floor
2. Bring your right knee forward, positioning it behind your right wrist with your right shin angled across the mat.
3. Extend your left leg straight back, keeping your left hip aligned with the mat.
4. Square your hips and align your right knee with your right hip.
5. Walk your hands forward, lowering your upper body toward the mat, and rest your forehead on your hands or a block if it feels comfortable.
6. Hold for several deep breaths, feeling the stretch in your right hip and groin.
7. Repeat on the other side.

Beginner's Tips:

- If you feel any discomfort in your front knee, place a blanket or block under your hip for added support
- Keep your back leg extended straight and avoid letting your hip sink.
- If you can't comfortably reach the floor, use props like blocks or blankets to support your forehead and chest.

Benefits:

- Deeply stretches the hip flexors and external rotators.
- Promotes flexibility in the hips and groin.
- Releases stress in the pelvic floor and lower back.
- Can help improve digestion and circulation.

Watch Out For:

- **Knee pain:** If you encounter any knee pain, alter the stance or come out of it.
- **Sacroiliac (SI) joint discomfort:** If you have any SI joint difficulties, proceed with caution or avoid this posture completely.
- **Overstretching:** Don't force the pose; go only as far as feels comfortable.

Variations:

1. **Reclining Pigeon Pose:** Lie on your back and raise your right ankle to your left thigh, just above your knee. Gently bring your left thigh closer to your chest by interlacing your fingers behind it.
2. **Figure Four Stretch:** Similar to Reclining Pigeon, except flex your right foot and gently press your right knee away from you.

Exercise 30

Happy Baby Pose (Ananda Balasana)

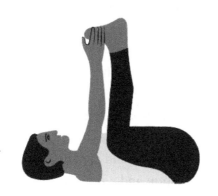

Steps:

1. Recline on your back and bring your legs up towards your chest.
2. Reach for the outer edges of your feet or ankles and gently pull them towards your armpits.
3. Ensure that your head and shoulders remain relaxed on the mat
4. Gently rock from side to side or hold the pose for a few breaths.

Beginner's Tips:

- If you can't reach your feet, use a strap or towel to assist the stretch.
- Keep your back flat on the mat and avoid arching your lower back.
- Relax your neck and shoulders.

Benefits:

- Gently stretch the inner thighs, groin, and hamstrings
- Promotes relaxation and release of tension in the pelvic floor muscles.
- Can help ease tension and anxiety.
- Improves digestion and circulation.

Watch Out For:

- **Neck strain:** Keep your neck neutral and avoid lifting your head off the mat.
- **Knee pain:** If you encounter any knee pain, change the pose or come out of it.

Variations:

1. **Happy Baby with legs wide:** Instead of raising your knees towards your armpits, let them fall open to the sides, producing a wider stretch.
2. **Happy Baby with one leg extended:** Extend one leg straight up towards the ceiling while holding the other leg in Happy Baby Pose.

Exercise 31

Wide-Legged Forward Fold (Prasarita Padottanasana)

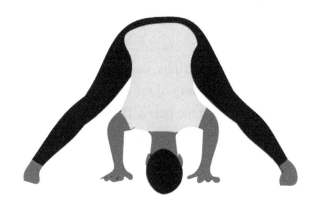

Steps:

1. Stand with your feet about 3-4 feet apart. Rotate your toes slightly inward and your heels slightly outward.
2. Inhale to lengthen your spine, then exhale and fold forward from your hips, keeping your back flat.
3. Rest your hands on the floor, on blocks, or on your shins
4. Release your head and neck towards the floor.
5. Hold for several breaths, feeling the stretch in your hamstrings and inner thighs.

Beginner's Tips:

- Bend your knees slightly if your hamstrings feel tight.
- Keep your back flat and avoid rounding your spine.
- If you can't reach the floor, use bricks under your hands for support.

Benefits:

- Stretches the hamstrings, calves, and inner thighs.
- Promotes lengthening of the spine.
- Releases stress in the pelvic floor and lower back.
- Calms the mind and relieves stress.

Watch Out For:

- **Rounding your back:** Keep your back flat, even if it means bending your knees.
- **Hamstring strain:** Don't force the stretch; go only as far as feels comfortable.

Variations:

1. **Wide-Legged Forward Fold with a chair:** Place your hands on a chair for support.
2. **Wide-Legged Forward Fold with a strap:** Loop a strap around your feet and grip onto it for support.

Exercise 32

Butterfly Pose (Baddha Konasana)

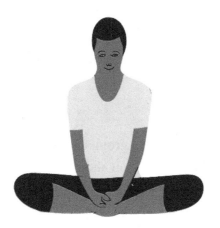

Steps:

1. Sit on the floor with your legs stretched out straight in front of you.
2. Bend your knees and bring the soles of your feet together, allowing your knees to fall wide to the sides.
3. Hold your feet with your hands and slowly bring them towards your pelvis.
4. Lengthen your spine and maintain your back straight.
5. Hold for several breaths, allowing your hips and groin to relax.

Beginner's Tips:

- If your hips feel tight, sit on a block or blanket to elevate your seat.
- Use props for support: Place blocks or blankets under your knees for comfort and to encourage relaxation.
- Avoid forcing your knees down; let gravity do the work.

Benefits:

- Opens the hips and groin, creating flexibility.
- Encourages relaxation and release of tension in the pelvic floor muscles.
- Improves circulation to the pelvic area.
- Can help alleviate period cramps and discomfort.

Watch Out For:

- **Knee pain:** If you encounter any knee pain, change the pose or come out of it.
- **Overstretching:** Avoid pulling your knees down; let gravity do the work.

Variations:

1. **Supported Butterfly Pose:** Place a bolster or blanket beneath your spine for additional support and comfort.
2. **Butterfly Pose with forward fold:** Gently fold forward from your hips, maintaining your back straight.

Exercise 33

Reclining Spinal Twist (Supta Jathara Parivartanasana)

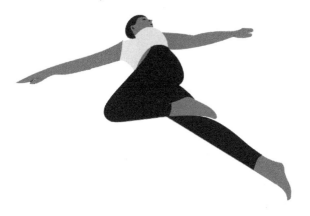

Steps:

1. Lie (Recline) on your back with your knees bent and feet flat on the floor.
2. Stretch your arms out to the sides in a T-shape, with your palms facing downward
3. Exhale and gently lower both knees to the right, keeping your shoulders pressed flat on the mat.
4. Rotate your head to the left, gazing over your left shoulder.
5. Hold this position for several breaths, then inhale and bring your knees back to the center.
6. Repeat on the other side.

Beginner's Tips:

- If your knees don't comfortably reach the floor, lay a block or blanket under them for support.
- Keep your shoulders relaxed and pressed into the mat.
- If you feel any strain in your neck, keep your head facing the ceiling.

Benefits:

- Gently stretch the spine, shoulders, and hips.
- Massages the abdominal organs, improving digestion.
- Enhances circulation and lymphatic flow.
- Reduces stress and tension in the pelvic floor and abdomen.

Watch out for:

- Forcing the twist: Go only as far as feels comfortable, avoiding any pain or strain.
- Lifting your shoulders off the mat: Keep your shoulders loose and planted.
- If you have any back, neck, or shoulder issues, visit a yoga instructor before attempting this posture.

Variations:

1. **The supine twist with a strap:** If your knees don't reach the floor, use a strap to gently guide them down.

2. **The supine twist with eagle legs:** Cross your right thigh over your left and wrap your right foot around your left calf for a deeper hip stretch.Supported

Exercise 34

Fish Pose (Matsyasana with supports)

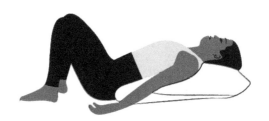

Steps:

1. Position a bolster or a rolled-up blanket lengthwise on your mat
2. Sit in front of the bolster with your knees bent and feet flat on the floor.
3. Gently drop your back onto the bolster, ensuring your head and neck are supported.
4. If needed, lay a block or blanket beneath your head for added support.
5. Extend your arms out to the sides, palms facing up, or rest them on your tummy.
6. Relax your entire body and breathe deeply.

7. Hold for 5-10 minutes.

Beginner's Tips:

- Adjust the height of the bolster or blankets to ensure your head and neck are adequately supported.
- If you feel any strain in your lower back, tuck a rolled-up towel under your knees.
- Close your eyes and focus on your breath to deepen your relaxation.

Benefits:

- Opens the chest and shoulders, encouraging deep breathing and lung capacity.
- Stretches the throat and neck muscles.
- Stimulates the thyroid and parathyroid glands.
- Promotes relaxation and stress reduction, indirectly benefitting pelvic floor health.

Watch out for:

- **Neck strain:** Ensure your head and neck are completely supported.
- **Lower back discomfort:** If you feel any tension, adjust the props or come out of the pose.

Variations:

1. **Supported Fish Pose using a block beneath your shoulder blades:** This might allow a deeper chest opening.

2. **Supported Fish Pose with legs extended:** If comfortable, extend your legs straight out in front of you.

Exercise 37

Legs up the Wall Pose with Strap (Viparita Karani with strap)

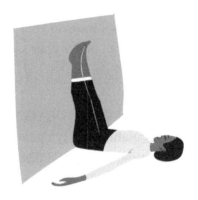

Steps:

1. Sit sideways against a wall, with your hip near to the wall.
2. Carefully lift your legs up the wall while reclining on the floor.
3. Position a yoga strap over your thighs, slightly above your knees, to help maintain your legs in position.
4. Place your arms by your sides with your palms facing up.
5. Close your eyes and let your entire body relax.

6. Hold for 5-10 minutes, breathing deeply and evenly.

Beginner's Tips:

- If your hamstrings feel tight, step slightly away from the wall or place a blanket under your hips for support.
- Adjust the tightness of the strap to provide comfort and stability.
- If you notice any soreness in your lower back, lay a little rolled-up cloth under your sacrum.

Benefits:

- Promotes relaxation and relieves weariness.
- Improves circulation and lymphatic drainage.
- Relieves swelling ankles and feet.
- Calms the mind and decreases stress, indirectly benefitting pelvic floor health.
- The strap gives additional support and helps hold the stance for longer durations.

Watch out for:

- **Neck strain:** If your neck feels strained, tuck a blanket or pillow under your head for support.
- **Discomfort in the lower back:** If you suffer any discomfort, modify your position or lay a towel under your sacrum.

- If you have any glaucoma or high blood pressure, see a healthcare practitioner before attempting this pose.

Variations:

1. **Legs-up-the-wall without a strap:** If you feel comfortable, you can practice the pose without the strap.
2. **Legs-up-the-wall with a bolster:** Place a bolster under your hips for more support and comfort.

Exercise 38

Corpse Pose (Savasana)

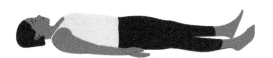

Steps:

1. Recline on your back with your legs extended and your arms by your sides, palms facing up. Close your eyes and allow your entire body to relax.
2. Release any tightness in your muscles and allow your breath to flow naturally.

3. Stay in this pose for five to ten minutes, focusing on deep relaxation and letting go of any thoughts or worries.

Beginner's Tips:

- If you feel any soreness in your lower back, tuck a little rolled-up towel or blanket under your knees.
- Cover yourself with a blanket to be warm and comfy.
- If your mind wanders, gently bring your attention back to your breath or the feelings in your body.

Benefits:

- Promotes profound relaxation and stress relief.
- Allows for total release of tension throughout the body, including the pelvic floor muscles.
- Improves sleep quality.
- Reduces anxiety and sadness.
- Boosts the immunological system.

Watch out for:

- **Falling asleep:** While it's typical to feel tired in Savasana, strive to stay awake and mindful of your breath and body sensations.
- **Discomfort:** If you suffer any discomfort, modify your position or utilize props for support.

Variations:

1. **Savasana with an eye pillow:** Place an eye cushion over your eyes to increase relaxation and block out light.

2. **Savasana with a blanket over your body:** This might help you feel more grounded and comfortable.

3. Listen to a guided meditation to enhance your relaxation and focus your attention.

Chapter 6

Balancing Poses: Enhancing Coordination and Control

Balance is both a physical and mental practice. As you challenge your coordination in these balancing poses, you're not just enhancing your physical stability, but also cultivating focus, patience, and control over your body. Each wobble is a reminder that balance is a journey, not a destination. Celebrate every small victory, and trust in your ability to find steadiness within

Exercise 39

Eagle Pose (Garudasana)

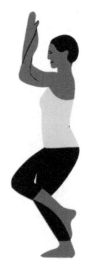

Steps:

1. Begin in Mountain Pose (Tadasana) with your feet set hip-width apart.
2. Bend your knees slightly and move your weight onto your left foot.
3. Cross your right thigh over your left thigh, hooking your right foot behind your left leg if feasible.
4. Wrap your right arm beneath your left arm, bending your elbows and bringing your hands together.
5. Lift your elbows to shoulder height and glance forward.
6. Hold for a few breaths, then release and repeat on the other side.

Beginner's Tips:

- If you can't wrap your foot around your calf, simply press the top of your foot against your lower thigh.
- If your arms don't bind, grasp onto your opposite shoulders or use a strap to link your hands.
- Focus on keeping your core engaged and your spine long.
- If you lose your equilibrium, simply release the stance and try again.

Benefits:

- Improves balance, attention, and coordination.

- Strengthens the legs, ankles, and core, especially the pelvic floor.
- Stretches the shoulders, upper back, and hips.
- Increases circulation and energy flow.

Watch out for:

- **Knee pain:** If you experience any knee pain, alter the stance or come out of it.
- **Ankle strain:** Avoid over-twisting your ankles.
- **Shoulder discomfort:** If your shoulders are tense, don't press the bind.

Variations:

1. **Eagle Pose with a chair:** Use a chair for assistance if balancing is problematic.
2. **Seated Eagle Pose:** Perform the arm bind while seated in a comfortable cross-legged position.

Exercise 40

Standing Hand to Big Toe Pose (Utthita Hasta Padangusthasana)

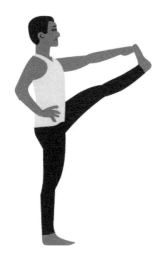

Steps:

1. Begin in Mountain Pose (Tadasana) with your feet hip-width apart.
2. Transfer your weight onto your left foot and bend your right knee.
3. Reach your right hand towards your right big toe, using a strap if needed.
4. Extend your right leg forward, maintaining it straight.
5. Activate your core and keep your back straight.
6. Hold for a few breaths, then switch and repeat on the other side.

Beginner's Tips:

- Keep your standing leg slightly bent if you're difficult to balance.
- Use a strap around your foot if you can't reach your big toe.
- Focus on stretching your spine and keeping your core engaged.

Benefits:

- Improves balance and coordination.
- Strengthens the legs, ankles, and core, especially the pelvic floor.
- Stretches the hamstrings and calves.
- Promotes focus and concentration.

Watch out for:

- Hyperextending your standing knee: Keep a modest bend in your standing knee.
- Rounding your back: Maintain a straight back and keep your core engaged.
- If you have any hamstring or groin issues, consult a yoga instructor before attempting this position.

Variations:

1. **Standing Hand to Big Toe Pose with a Chair:** Use a chair for support if balancing is problematic.

2. **Standing Hand to Big Toe Pose with a bent knee:** Keep your lifted knee bent if you can't straighten your leg entirely.

Exercise 41

Warrior III with Block (Virabhadrasana III with block)

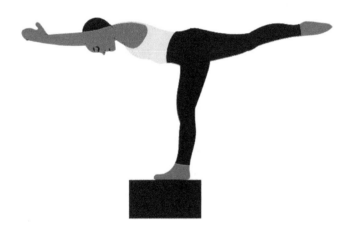

Steps:

1. Start in Mountain Pose (Tadasana).
2. Step your right foot back and lay a yoga block under your right heel.
3. Raise your left leg so it's parallel to the floor, hinging forward at your hips.

4. Keep your back straight and core engaged.
5. Extend your arms forward with your palms facing each other
6. Hold for several breaths, then exchange sides.

Beginner's Tips:

- Use a wall or chair for support if balancing is problematic.
- Keep your focus on a fixed spot in front of you to assist in maintaining balance.
- Focus on using your core and pelvic floor muscles for stability.

Benefits:

- Improves balance and coordination.
- Strengthens the legs, ankles, and core, especially the pelvic floor.
- Stretches the hamstrings and calves.
- The block offers extra difficulty, requiring greater core and pelvic floor activation.

Watch out for:

- **Arching your back:** Maintain a straight back to avoid tension.
- **Dropping your lifted leg:** Keep your lifted leg parallel to the floor.

Variations:

1. Warrior III without a block: Practice the standard Warrior III stance without the block for a less intense alternative.
2. Warrior III with hands on hips: If balancing is problematic, lay your hands on your hips.

Exercise 42

Dancer Pose (Natarajasana)

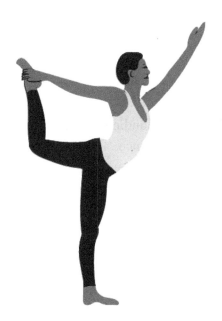

Steps:

1. Stand in Mountain Pose (Tadasana).
2. Bend your right knee and reach your right hand back to hold your right foot or ankle.
3. Lift your right foot towards the ceiling, maintaining your left leg straight and your core engaged.
4. Extend your left arm forward, reaching toward the horizon.
5. Gaze ahead or slightly upwards.
6. Hold for a few breaths, then release and repeat on the other side.

Beginner's Tips:

- Use a strap around your foot if you can't reach it with your hand.
- Keep your standing leg slightly bent if you're difficult to balance.
- Concentrate on elongating your spine and keeping your chest open.

Benefits:

- Improves balance, flexibility, and coordination.
- Strengthens the legs, ankles, and core, especially the pelvic floor.
- Stretches the shoulders, chest, and hip flexors.
- Promotes focus and concentration.

Watch out for:

- **Hyperextending your standing knee:** Keep a modest bend in your standing knee.
- **Rounding your back:** Maintain a straight back and keep your core engaged

Variations:

1. **Dancer Pose with a chair:** Use a chair for assistance if balancing is problematic.
2. **Modified Dancer Pose:** Keep your lifted knee bent and grasp onto your shin instead of your foot.

Exercise 43

Half Moon Pose (Ardha Chandrasana)

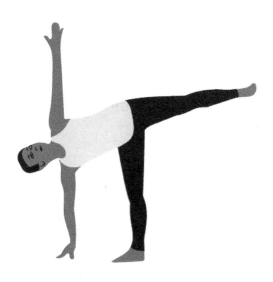

Steps:

1. Begin in Triangle Pose (Trikonasana) with your right foot forward.
2. Bend your right knee slightly and bring your right hand on the floor or a block about a foot in front of your right foot.
3. Shift your weight onto your right foot and elevate your left leg parallel to the floor.
4. Extend your left arm towards the ceiling, keeping your palm facing down.
5. Gaze up towards your left hand.
6. Hold for several breaths, then exchange sides.

Beginner's Tips:

- Use a block under your bottom hand for support if needed.
- Maintain a straight back and keep your core engaged
- If balancing is problematic, practice near a wall for support.

Benefits:

- Strengthens the legs, ankles, and core, especially the pelvic floor.
- Improves balance, coordination, and focus.
- Stretches the hamstrings, calves, groin, and spine.
- Opens the chest and shoulders.

Watch out for:

- **Hyperextending your standing knee:** Keep a modest bend in your standing knee.
- **Collapsing in your chest:** Keep your chest open and your top arm stretching towards the ceiling.
- **Neck strain:** If your neck feels strained, maintain your gaze forward instead of gazing up.

Variations:

1. **Half Moon Pose with a Block:** Place a block under your bottom hand for support.
2. **Half Moon Pose with a wall:** Practice along a wall for support and stability.

Exercise 44

Crow Pose (Bakasana)

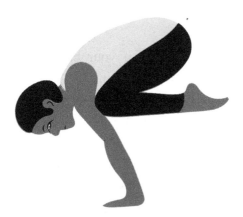

Steps:

1. Start in a squat stance with your feet hip-width apart and your knees bent deeply.
2. Place your hands shoulder-width apart on the carpet in front of you, fingers extended wide.
3. Lean forward and position your knees on the backs of your upper arms, close to your armpits.
4. Shift your weight forward, lifting your feet off the floor one at a time.
5. Gaze forward and engage your core and pelvic floor muscles for stability.
6. Hold for a few breaths, then gradually lower your feet back to the floor.

Beginner's Tips:

- Practice alongside a wall for support if needed.
- Place a block under your feet to assist you lift them off the floor.
- Focus on rounding your back and moving your navel towards your spine.
- Engage your pelvic floor muscles to help maintain balance and control

Benefits:

- Strengthens the arms, wrists, core, and pelvic floor.
- Improves balance, coordination, and focus.
- Builds confidence and overcomes fear.

Watch out for:

- **Wrist trouble:** If you feel wrist pain, alter the pose or use wrist wraps for support.
- **Face planting:** If you feel like you're going to fall forward, duck your chin to your chest to protect your face.
- If you have any wrist, shoulder, or back issues, consult a yoga instructor before attempting this posture.

Variations:

1. **Crow Pose with a block:** Place a block beneath your feet for support.
2. **Side Crow Pose:** Balance on one arm and the outer edge of the same foot, stacking your feet or staggering them for extra stability.

Exercise 45

Side Plank Pose (Vasisthasana)

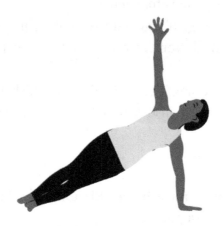

Steps:

1. Start in Plank Pose (Phalakasana).
2. Shift your weight onto your right hand and the outer border of your right foot.
3. Stack your left foot on top of your right foot or place it slightly in front for greater support.
4. Reach your left arm towards the ceiling, keeping your palm facing down.
5. Gaze up towards your left hand or keep your neck neutral.
6. Hold for several breaths, then exchange sides.

Beginner's Tips:

- If balancing is challenging, lower your bottom knee to the floor for support.

- Keep your core engaged and your hips lifted.
- Avoid letting your hips drop or your shoulders slump.

Benefits:

- Strengthens the obliques, core, arms, and pelvic floor.
- Improves balance and stability.
- Stretches the wrists and hamstrings.

Watch out for:

- **Wrist trouble:** If you feel wrist pain, alter the pose or use wrist wraps for support.
- **Shoulder collapse:** Keep your shoulders packed and prevent letting them round forward.
- **Hip sagging:** Keep your hips elevated and your body in a straight line.

Variations:

1. **Side Plank with a block:** Position a block under your bottom hand for additional support.
2. **Side Plank with leg lift:** Lift your upper leg towards the ceiling for added difficulty.

Chapter 7

Restorative Poses: Deep Relaxation for Pelvic Health

Rest is a powerful tool for healing and rejuvenation. In these restorative poses, give yourself permission to slow down, breathe deeply, and sink into a state of profound relaxation. This chapter is your opportunity to restore not only your pelvic health but also your overall well-being. Embrace this time as a gift to yourself, knowing that relaxation is just as important as strength in your practice.

Exercise 46

Supported Reclining Butterfly Pose (Supta Baddha Konasana with props)

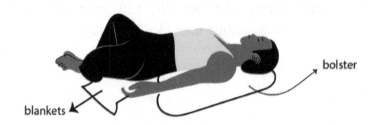

Steps:

1. Gather props: You'll need a bolster, one or two blankets, and possibly, an eye pillow.
2. Place the bolster lengthwise on your mat.
3. Sit in front of the bolster, bringing the soles of your feet together and allowing your knees to fall open to the sides.
4. Place blankets beneath your knees for support, ensuring they are comfortable and enable your legs to rest entirely.
5. Gently drop your back onto the bolster, adjusting it so that it supports your entire spine.
6. If desired, place an eye pillow over your eyes.
7. Relax your entire body and place your arms at your sides with your palms facing up.
8. Hold for 5-10 minutes, breathing deeply and evenly.

Beginner's Tips:

- Use props generously: The more support you have, the deeper the relaxation you'll experience.
- If your hips are tight, tuck additional blankets or blocks beneath your outer thighs.
- If your neck feels strained, lay a little rolled-up blanket beneath your neck for support.

Benefits:

- Deepens the relaxation of the pelvic floor, groin, and inner thighs.
- Encourages the release of tension and stress.
- Improves circulation to the pelvic area.
- Can help alleviate period cramps and discomfort.
- Promotes deep breathing and relaxation.

Watch out for:

- **Knee pain:** If you suffer any knee pain, modify the props or come out of the pose.
- **Neck strain:** Ensure your neck is comfortably supported.

Variations:

1. **Supported Reclining Butterfly Pose with a strap:** If your knees don't comfortably fall open, wrap a strap around your thighs to gently support them.
2. **Supported Reclining Butterfly Pose with essential oils**: Add a few drops of lavender or chamomile essential oil to your bolster or tissue near your face to improve relaxation.

Exercise 47

Supported Bridge Pose (Setu Bandhasana with props)

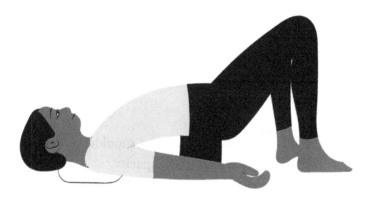

Steps:

1. Gather props: Two or three blankets and a yoga block are required.
2. Lie on your back with your legs bent and feet flat on the floor, hip-width apart.
3. Place the block under your sacrum, adjusting the height as needed for comfort.
4. Place a folded blanket beneath your shoulders and neck for support.
5. Relax your entire body and place your arms at your sides with your palms facing up.
6. Hold for 5-10 minutes, breathing deeply and evenly.

Beginner's Tips:

- Start with the lowest height on the block and progressively increase as you feel comfortable.
- If you feel any strain in your neck, move the blanket under your shoulders or use an additional blanket for support.
- If your feet turn out, insert a block between your thighs to help keep them parallel.

Benefits:

- Gently expands the chest and shoulders, facilitating deep breathing and lung capacity.
- Stretches the hip flexors and thighs.
- Encourages relaxation and stress reduction, indirectly benefitting pelvic floor health.
- Improves circulation and lymphatic drainage.

Watch out for

- **Neck strain:** Ensure your neck is adequately supported and comfortable.
- **Lower back discomfort:** If you feel any tension, adjust the props or come out of the pose.

Variations:

1. **Supported Bridge Pose with a bolster:** Place a bolster lengthwise under your spine for increased support and comfort.

2. **Supported Bridge Pose with an eye pillow:** Add an eye pillow to increase relaxation and deepen the pose.

Exercise 48

Legs on a Chair Pose

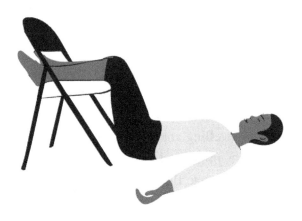

Steps:

1. For support, lean a chair up against a wall.
2. Place your hips just a few inches from the wall while lying on your back.
3. Put your heels up against the wall as you extend your legs up it.
4. Put your arms down by your sides, palms up.
5. Close your eyes and unwind throughout your body.

6. Hold for 5-10 minutes, breathing deeply and evenly.

Beginner's Tips:

- If your hamstrings feel tight, step slightly away from the wall or place a blanket under your hips for support.
- If you notice any soreness in your lower back, lay a little rolled-up cloth under your sacrum.

Benefits:

- Promotes relaxation and relieves weariness.
- Improves circulation and lymphatic drainage.
- Relieves swelling ankles and feet.
- Calms the mind and decreases stress, indirectly benefitting pelvic floor health.
- Encourages relaxation of the pelvic floor muscles.

Watch out for:

- **Neck strain:** If your neck feels strained, tuck a blanket or pillow under your head for support.
- **Discomfort in the lower back:** If you suffer any discomfort, modify your position or lay a towel under your sacrum.

Variations:

1. **Legs on a Chair Pose with a bolster:** Place a bolster beneath your knees for increased support and comfort

2. **Legs on a Chair position with an eye cushion:** Add an eye pillow to improve relaxation and deepen the position.

Exercise 49

Constructive Rest Pose

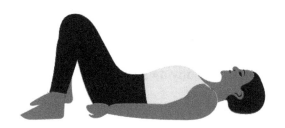

Steps:

1. Lie on your back with your legs bent and feet flat on the floor, hip-width apart.
2. Keep your arms at your sides, palms up.
3. Close your eyes and relax any tension in your muscles.
4. Allow your breath to flow naturally and note the rise and fall of your abdomen.
5. Stay in this pose for five to ten minutes, focusing on deep relaxation and letting go of any thoughts or worries.

Beginner's Tips:

- If you feel any soreness in your lower back, tuck a little rolled-up towel or blanket under your knees.
- You can also lay a blanket under your head for additional support and comfort.

Benefits:

- Promotes deep relaxation of the entire body, especially the pelvic floor muscles.
- Reduces tension and anxiety.
- Improves sleep quality.
- Enhances bodily awareness and mindfulness.

Watch out for:

- **Falling asleep:** While it's typical to feel tired in this pose, try to stay awake and mindful of your breath and body sensations.
- **Discomfort:** If you suffer any discomfort, modify your position or utilize props for support.

Variations:

1. **Constructive Rest Pose with a bolster:** Place a bolster beneath your knees for increased support and comfort.
2. **Constructive Rest Pose with an eye cushion:** Add an eye pillow to increase relaxation and block out light.

Exercise 50

Supported Child's Pose (Balasana with supports)

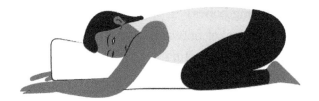

Steps:

1. Gather props: You'll need a bolster or a few folded blankets.
2. Bring your big toes together while on your knees, letting your knees spread widely apart.
3. Place the bolster or blankets lengthwise in front of you.
4. Fold forward from your hips, resting your torso on the bolster or blankets.
5. Turn your head to one side and rest your forehead on the bolster or blankets.
6. Extend your arms beside your body, palms facing up.
7. Relax your entire body and breathe deeply.

8. Hold for 5-10 minutes, adjusting the direction of your head halfway through.

Beginner's Tips:

- Adjust the height of the bolster or blankets to ensure your forehead and torso are comfortably supported.
- If your hips are tight, tuck a rolled-up blanket under your sitting bones.
- Place a blanket between your thighs and calves if your knees are hurting.

Benefits:

- Gently stretch the back, hips, and shoulders.
- Promotes relaxation and release of tension in the pelvic floor and hips.
- Calms the mind and relieves stress.
- Improves digestion and circulation.

Watch out for:

- **Knee pain:** If you encounter any knee pain, change the pose or come out of it.
- **Neck strain:** Ensure your neck is comfortably supported and neutral.

Variations:

1. **Supported Child's Pose with a block under your forehead:** If your forehead doesn't comfortably

reach the bolster, place a block beneath it for support.

2. **Supported Child's Pose with arms extended overhead:** Extend your arms aloft and rest them on the bolster or blankets for a moderate shoulder stretch.

Exercise 51

Yoga Nidra

Steps:

1. Find a tranquil and comfortable spot where you won't be interrupted.
2. Lie on your back in Savasana (Corpse Pose) with your legs extended and arms by your sides, palms facing up.

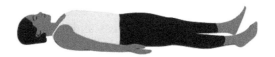

3. Close your eyes and begin to follow the guided directions of a Yoga Nidra tape or teacher.

4. The practice often comprises methodical relaxing of the body, breath awareness, and visualization exercises.

5. Allow yourself to fully surrender to the experience and let go of any ideas or fears.

Beginner's Tips:

- Choose a Yoga Nidra recording or teacher that resonates with you.
- Make sure you're warm and comfortable, using blankets or props as needed.
- Set aside adequate time for the practice, often 20-30 minutes.
- If your mind wanders, gently bring your attention back to the instructions or your breath.

Benefits:

- Induces deep relaxation and promotes healing on physical, mental, and emotional levels.
- Reduces stress, anxiety, and insomnia.
- Improves focus and concentration.
- Enhances self-awareness and intuition.
- Indirectly helps pelvic floor health by encouraging overall relaxation and stress reduction.

Watch out for:

- Falling asleep: While it's usual to feel tired during Yoga Nidra, strive to stay awake and conscious of the practice.

- If you have any mental health concerns, see a healthcare expert before practicing Yoga Nidra.

Exercise 52

Savasana with Eye Pillow

Steps:

1. Lie on your back in Savasana (Corpse Pose) with your legs extended and arms by your sides, palms facing up.
2. Place an eye pillow over your eyes.
3. Release any tightness in your muscles and allow your breath to flow naturally.
4. Stay in this pose for five to ten minutes, focusing on deep relaxation and letting go of any thoughts or worries.

Beginner's Tips:

- If you feel any soreness in your lower back, tuck a little rolled-up towel or blanket under your knees.
- Cover yourself with a blanket to be warm and comfy.
- If your mind wanders, gently bring your attention back to your breath or the feelings in your body.

Benefits:

- Promotes profound relaxation and stress relief.

- Allows for total release of tension throughout the body, including the pelvic floor muscles.
- Improves sleep quality.
- Reduces anxiety and sadness.
- Boosts the immunological system.
- The eye pillow enhances relaxation by blocking out light and promoting a deeper sense of calm.

Watch out for:

- **Falling asleep:** While it's typical to feel tired in Savasana, strive to stay awake and mindful of your breath and body sensations.
- **Discomfort:** If you suffer any discomfort, modify your position or utilize props for support.

Variations:

1. **Savasana with a blanket over your body:** This might help you feel more grounded and comfortable.
2. **Savasana with aromatherapy:** Add a few drops of lavender or chamomile essential oil on a tissue near your head to increase relaxation.

Chapter 8: Bonus

Daily Routines: Short Practices for Busy Lives

Consistency is key to lasting change. These short, daily routines are designed to fit seamlessly into your busy life, offering you the benefits of pelvic floor yoga without overwhelming your schedule. Even a few minutes of mindful practice each day can make a significant difference. Commit to these routines, and watch how small, consistent efforts lead to lasting improvements in your strength, flexibility, and overall health.

Morning Pelvic Floor Activation:

Start your day by lying in bed and practicing 5-10 rounds of Kegel exercises, coordinating with your breath. This helps awaken and tone your pelvic floor muscles.

Chair Yoga Break:

During a work break, try seated Cat-Cow, twists, or pelvic tilts. These simple movements improve circulation, reduce tension, and promote pelvic floor awareness.

Mindful Walking:

While walking, focus on engaging your pelvic floor muscles with each step. This integrates pelvic floor awareness into daily activities.

Evening Wind-Down Flow:

Before bed, practice a short sequence of gentle poses like Child's Pose, Reclining Bound Angle Pose, and Legs-up-the-Wall Pose to release tension and prepare for restful sleep.

Breath Awareness Meditation:

Take 5-10 minutes to sit quietly and observe your breath. Notice how your pelvic floor responds to your inhales and exhales, fostering a deeper mind-body connection.

Quick Core Activation:

Perform a few rounds of Plank Pose or Bird Dog during a commercial break or while waiting for your coffee to brew. These exercises strengthen your core, indirectly supporting your pelvic floor.

Restorative Yoga Before Bed:

Practice a few restorative poses like Supported Child's Pose or Legs on a Chair Pose before bed to calm your nervous system and promote relaxation in your pelvic floor muscles.

Pelvic Floor Contractions During Daily Tasks:

While brushing your teeth, washing dishes, or waiting in line, practice a few sets of Kegel exercises. This helps build strength and endurance throughout the day.

Yoga Nidra for Deep Relaxation:

If you have 20-30 minutes, try a Yoga Nidra session. This guided meditation promotes deep relaxation, benefiting both your mental and physical health, including your pelvic floor.

Mindful Shower or Bath:

During your shower or bath, take a few moments to focus on your pelvic floor muscles. Practice gentle contractions and releases, visualizing the muscles lifting and relaxing.

28-Day Pelvic Floor Yoga Challenge: Reclaim Your Power

Week	Day	Focus	Poses & Practices
Week 1: Foundations & Connection	1	Introduction & Gentle Flow	Pelvic Floor Intro (Reading), Cat-Cow (pg. 35), Pelvic Tilts (pg. 37)
	2	Core Awareness	Deep Core Exercises, Plank Pose (pg. 19)
	3	Gentle Flow & Release	Child's Pose to Downward-Facing Dog (pg. 39), Seated Spinal Twist (pg. 46)
	4	Core Strength	Bird Dog (pg. 21), Bridge Pose (pg. 23)
	5	Restorative	Legs-up-the-Wall Pose (pg. 51), Savasana with Eye Pillow (118)
	6	Gentle Flow	Standing Forward Fold to Halfway Lift (pg. 42), Supine Spinal Twist (pg. 48)
	7	REST	

Week 2: Building Strength & Stability	8	Core Power	Boat Pose (pg. 25), Chair Pose (pg. 27)
	9	Standing Strength	Warrior II (pg. 53), Triangle Pose (pg. 55)
	10	Deep Core & Stretch	Extended Side Angle Pose (pg. 58), Reclining Bound Angle Pose (pg. 67)
	11	Balance & Focus	Tree Pose (pg. 62), Mountain Pose with Arm Circles (pg. 44)
	12	Restorative	Supported Reclining Butterfly Pose (pg. 105), Yoga Nidra (pg. 116)
	13	Core Challenge	Warrior III (pg. 30), High Lunge (pg. 60)
	14	REST	

Week 3: Flexibility & Release	15	Hip Openers	Pigeon Pose (pg. 71), Happy Baby Pose (pg. 74)
	16	Hamstring & Spine	Wide-Legged Forward Fold (pg. 76), Reclining Spinal Twist (pg. 80)
	17	Deep Stretch & Release	Butterfly Pose (pg. 78), Supported Bridge Pose (pg. 108)
	18	Balance & Core	Goddess Pose (pg. 32), Bridge Pose with Block (pg. 64)
	19	Restorative	Legs on a Chair Pose (pg. 110), Constructive Rest Pose (pg. 112)
	20	Grounding Flow	Squat Pose (pg. 69), Fish Pose with supports (pg. 82)
	21	REST	

Week 4: Integration & Empowerment	22	Challenge & Balance	Eagle Pose (pg. 89), Standing Hand to Big Toe Pose (pg. 92)
	23	Full Body Flow	Warrior III with Block (pg. 94), Dancer Pose (pg. 96)
	24	Core & Hip Flexor Release	Half Moon Pose (pg. 98), Supported Child's Pose (pg. 114)
	25	Deep Core & Balance	Crow Pose (pg. 100), Side Plank Pose (pg. 103)
	26	Restorative & Integration	Legs up the Wall Pose with Strap (pg. 84), Corpse Pose (pg. 86)
	27	Celebrate Your Progress!	Choose your favorite poses
	28	REST & Reflect	

A Letter from the Author

TO THE WOMEN WHO HAVE CHOSEN THIS BOOK AS A COMPANION ON THEIR JOURNEY TO PELVIC HEALTH AND WELL-BEING,

Congratulations on taking this empowering step towards reclaiming your strength, vitality, and connection with your body.

Whether you're a **new mother** navigating the postpartum landscape, a woman embracing the changes of **menopause**, or **simply seeking** to deepen your understanding of your pelvic floor, know that you are not alone.

This book is more than a collection of poses; it's an invitation to cultivate self-compassion, embrace your feminine power, and discover the transformative potential of yoga.

May each page **inspire** you to listen to your body's wisdom, honor its unique needs, and celebrate its inherent strength.

Remember, progress is not linear, and there is no "perfect" practice. Embrace the journey, celebrate your victories, and be kind to yourself along the way.

You are capable, you are resilient, and you are worthy of vibrant health and well-being.

With love and light,

Mandy Norris

Made in the USA
Las Vegas, NV
15 December 2024

14343768R00075